Sleep Training

Baby Sleep Training for Essential Rest and Peace of Mind

SARAH RENE

CONTENTS

1   Introduction   1

2   How Much Sleep Does Your Baby Need?   3

3   What Are The Signs My Baby Is Sleepy?   5

4   Basic Sleeping Facts   7.

5   Setting Up The Crib   9

6   How To Choose The Right Accessories   11

7   Sleeping Safety And SIDS   12

8   Tried And True Methods   15

9   Creating A Sleeping Plan   20

10   Do's And Do Not's   22

11   FAQ   24

12   Conclusion   26

13   Additional Resources   27

INTRODUCTION

Being a new mom or dad can really be tough. You are expected to do everything and more for your baby while running on just a few hours of sleep. Before this wonderful addition came into your life, you probably heard about how tired you would be, but nothing really prepares you for what you are going to experience. It's a zoo, but it is so worth it that you would be willing to go through hell and back to make everything okay.

As a parent, you lay up beside your son or daughter to hear his or her breathing. You listen to sounds of movement or waking. However, while you are doing this, you are also losing precious hours for yourself – so what can you do about it?

The best approach to getting yourself a restful night of sleep is to ensure that your baby is also resting peacefully and safely. To do this, you will not only have to ensure that your baby falls asleep safely, but also stays asleep and is safe in his or her environment. After all, humans can sense danger, which can inhibit sleep.

In this book, we will talk about different techniques that will help you to get your baby to sleep peacefully – resulting in a much happier baby, and therefore, a much happier mom and dad. Other things that you can do will include the presence of comfort objects, playing music, co-sleeping, and the good old fashioned crying it out method.

You will also learn about things that you can do before your baby is born, like setting up a crib that is comfortable for the baby. Purchasing books or mobiles will help them, and even strategically setting up the nursery so that you can move around your house freely, but get to your baby in a time of need.

We will also talk about the science of sleeping, and focus on just how much sleep your baby needs. While it will seem like he or she isn't sleeping all that much, you will be surprised at just how much there actually is – it is just filled with many little breaks.

This book will walk you through some of the most essential parts of sleeping, but also help you to make a sleeping plan that will work for your entire family. Though every baby is different, there are a few different methods that you will be able to do to help encourage your baby to sleep, keep him sleeping, and even develop the skills that he will need for the rest of his life.

After all, a Harvard education and an excellent job all start with being fresh and ready to take on the world in the morning.

So what are you waiting for? Whether you are a new parent that is having trouble getting your baby to sleep, a veteran parent that is thinking about moving your toddler to a different sleep plan, or you are still expecting your first born and just want to prepare for the rest of your life, this is a great place to start your journey toward a more fulfilling, restful night.

HOW MUCH SLEEP DOES YOUR BABY NEED?

Now, the important thing to know is that each baby is different and these aren't necessarily "hard and fast" rules of sleeping. However, these are guidelines that will help you to determine an appropriate waking and sleeping time for your child. To make it easier and more concise, I've broken it down by the most important guideline: Age.

1-4 weeks old will need 15-16 hours of sleep per day.

Now that might seem like a lot, but newborns will typically sleep anywhere from 15 to 18 hours a day! However, they do this in shorter bursts of time, about 2-4 hours before they wake again. Babies who were premature will likely sleep more, and babies who are colicky will sleep less.

Newborns do not have something called circadian rhythms, or a natural body clock that tells them that light means wake and dark means sleep. This also means that they don't have a sleeping pattern, which can be frustrating. Thankfully, they seem to develop one relatively quickly.

1-4 months old will need 14-15 hours of sleep per day.

At around 6 weeks, your baby will start to become a regular sleeper, so long as you encourage that behavior. He will also be able to sleep for longer periods of time, often sleeping for 4-6 hours before waking. You will likely see the development of circadian rhythms during this period as well, ending your nightlong struggle to get your baby to sleep.

4-12 months old will need 14-16 hours of sleep per day.

There isn't a change in length here, and for a good reason. These numbers are ideal – it is far more likely that your infant will get about 12 hours of sleep a day. Your baby should be able to communicate a little more by the end of this stage, and should be developing habits. One of those habits is that his sleeping patterns will finally even out and he can wake and sleep at similar times.

Your baby should still have 2-3 naps per day at this stage, tapering out to two toward the 7-month mark. Most doctors will recommend a mid-morning nap at around 9 a.m. that lasts for about an hour (or adjust for your favorite morning talk show, like many parents do) and another nap that is just in time for dinner preparation, or around 4 p.m. This nap shouldn't last more than an hour as well, or he might not be tired in a few hours for bedtime.

1 to 3-year old should get 12-14 hours of sleep per day.
As your child is aging, naps will be harder to encourage, but that doesn't mean you shouldn't. Most toddlers will only get 10 hours of sleep per day, so you should encourage at least another nap in there somewhere. Many people suggest using lunchtime and then naptime as a routine that his body will get used to. As long as the rest occurs midday, you can let him sleep for as long as he would like (but not over 3.5 hours).

This sleeping schedule will keep you on track if you put him to bed anywhere from 7 to 9 p.m. and wake up anywhere from 6 to 8 a.m.

So how long should my baby sleep?
One again, these aren't hard and fast rules that you have to obey to have a baby that is well rested. You will need to feel out how much sleep your baby needs and whether or not he is tired. Work around your schedule as well – if you work a different shift, adjust the sleep how you like it. Just aim for those numbers!

WHAT ARE THE SIGNS MY BABY IS SLEEPY?

Babies need their sleep and knowing when your child is ready for that sleep will ensure that you too are going to get sleep. A regular schedule starts with understanding how and when your baby is tired. How can you do that? Well, once again it really depends on the child, but there are some basic signs that he or she is ready:

Watch How He Behaves
Actions are the easiest way to see how your baby behaves. Many babies will do similar things to what adults do: yawn, rub at their eyes, or start to drop their head. Other babies will suck on their fingers or fists. You will have to watch to know exactly what your baby will do, so pay attention!

Crying and Noises
Babies cry whenever they aren't happy, and that could include when they are tired and cranky. If your baby is crying a lot and he isn't wet or hungry, then you might want to try to put him to sleep. However, if he gets to the point that he is overtired, you might have some trouble.

Alertness
When your baby is tired, you will notice a distinct change in alertness. Since most children that have trouble sleeping can't really communicate, you will have to circle back around to their activity level. If they aren't paying attention to toys, television, food, or you, the chances are that they are quite tired.

Time of the Day
If your baby has a schedule (which he should once you are finished with this book), then you will be able to predict when he starts to get sleep.

Every day, it should happen around the same time. For younger babies, it can occur after events – for instance, they may get tired after going on a walk or being fed.

Some babies are different!
Some kids will give you different signs, even if they are within the same family. Think about how different your sleeping signs were from someone else in your family. Look for the subtle clues, especially a change in activity level and alertness, as those are often the first signs. Timing should really be your #1 indicator, especially if you are able to get him on a sleeping schedule.

Remember that "looking tired" isn't always the response either – listen to them as well!

Sticking to a schedule is important for your baby, especially if he has a difficult time sleeping. Children yearn for order and patterns. If at all possible, try to avoid any activities that will interrupt your baby's sleep schedule on any given day.

Another thing to be on the lookout for is if your baby is reaching for something called a comfort object. We will talk more about those later, but it is important to note that if your child is reaching for it, you have definitely got a sleepy baby on your hands.

If your baby has a regular babysitter (especially if it is grandparents) or is in daycare and has to sleep on a schedule that relates to the other kids in the school, your best bet is to continue that same schedule when they're at home, too. Consistency is the key!

BASIC SLEEPING FACTS

These facts really didn't fit into any of the other sections of the book, but they are important for you to note so that you can truly help your baby get to sleep. Try to remember these as you are reading the rest of the book, as they will help you to make different decisions about your baby and his/her sleeping patterns.

Fact 1: Babies have shorter sleeping cycles than adults do.

Have you ever wondered why babies wake up so often, even when they haven't slept for a long time? It is because they don't have the same sleep cycles! Babies will move from light sleep (REM) to deep sleep (NREM) about every hour or so. They wake up during that REM stage, and sometimes they will stay awake. Often, they will go right back to sleep without even realizing it – those are the good nights.

Fact 2: Just because a baby has his eyes closed, that doesn't mean he is asleep.

We always close our eyes when we act like we are sleeping, but in reality fluttering eyes is a sign of sleep. Your baby is still in REM stage then, however. You should wait until your baby is completely limp and isn't fluttering his eyelids before you put him down. If you don't wait, you risk waking him up.

Fact 3: Babies sleep so lightly for a very important reason.

Babies sleep lightly because they need food to survive. If they slept too deeply, they wouldn't be able to wake up when they are hungry and demand that they are fed. It is an evolutionary tick that we haven't quite worked out yet, but it holds significance and a bond with mom (and dad) that cannot be broken.

Fact 4: Babies need sleep so that they can develop.

Babies are so tired all the time because they are constantly growing and developing. From language skills to knee caps, all of the growing your baby is doing is definitely wearing him down all day long. If your baby doesn't get the right amount of sleep, you could be doing damage.

Fact 5: The better your baby sleeps during the day, the better he will sleep at night.

Many people think that giving your baby too many naps will mean that he won't sleep at night. In reality, a baby who is well rested will go to sleep more easily and sleep better at night than a baby who doesn't have the practice.

Fact 6: Darkness is important.

We have already talked about the importance of circadian rhythms, but here it is again. You should help your baby distinguish between night and day so that his or her body can release the appropriate levels of melatonin, which is the hormone that helps induce sleep.

SETTING THE CRIB

Even though it will feel like your baby falls asleep more in your arms than he does in his bed, it is still important to give him a great place to rest his head. There are differences between his bed and your bed that will make all the difference.

There are various things that you should and should not put into your baby's bed for safety reasons and practicality reasons. Think about those fluffy pillows you see on beds in movies and on television – are they actually practical or are they just going to go on the floor at night?

In reality, your baby's bed should feel like a safe haven for him, but also be comfortable enough so that sleep comes (and stays) easily.

Of course, that doesn't mean that you can't add some of your own flavors to the bedding, but you might want to keep things to a minimum.

A Basic List of What You'll Need for Your Baby's Crib

Fitted Sheets: this is truly the only thing a crib really needs if you are going to go bare bones. Check for sheets that are comfortable and snuggly, and go a little bit higher in your budget if you can. Also, make sure that the sheets you buy fit a crib mattress – most are standard size, but some will vary depending on where you buy it.

Waterproof Mattress Pads: no matter how much you spend on your mattress, you will want to protect it. A mattress pad will make everything nice and easy to clean up when you have leaks…which you will.

Anti-Allergen Cases: Your little one is still young, but dust mites and other airborne allergens are no joke. An anti-allergen casing goes over the entire mattress to help protect against not only dust mites, but also bed bugs. You can even get them waterproof so that you are covering all of your bases.

Bumpers: While many people think these are only to make the crib cuter, they actually serve a purpose. They keep your baby from slipping through the rails or banging a body part on them. They also just give a little bit of warmth. However, when your baby starts to crawl and climb, you might want to get rid of them!

Bed Skirts: Crib skirts are a great way to add some decoration to the crib without going over the top. It is also a good way to cover up some of the under bed storage you might have going on – just make sure that the skirt is long enough to cover all of the different setting that you may use, as the skirt moves with the mattress.

Notice that we didn't say a need for a pillow or a blanket. That's because you will either swaddle your baby or let him go without. You want to avoid putting anything in the crib that will potentially cover your baby's face while he is sleeping.

HOW TO CHOOSE THE RIGHT ACCESSORIES

When you are picking accessories, there are a few things that you should look for:

A good, tight fit: Just like with the blankets, your sheets and pads should fit snugly so that they don't come up.

Machine washable: Things get pretty dirty in those cribs, especially when baby starts to learn how to take off his own diaper.

Healthy: You've already read about how much time a baby spends sleeping in the first few years of life, so you want to make sure that what you buy is safe. It is a good idea to go toward organic sheets that are "Oeko-Tex Certified" which means that they weren't soaked in formaldehyde.

Sleep positioners. Keep your baby in the recommended position—on his back—with these bumpers that are placed next to the hips: the bumpers keep your baby from rolling onto his front accidentally but should not be used once he starts rolling over on purpose.

SLEEPING SAFETY AND SIDS

Most parents will admit that their biggest fear is that they will put their baby to sleep one night only for something to go wrong in the middle of the night. SIDS or Sudden Infant Death Syndrome occurs when a baby younger than 12 months dies when he is sleeping without a clear sign or warning.

Truthfully, there isn't a 100% way to prevent SIDS, but there are a lot of different things you can do to lower the risk. Here are just a few things you can do to make sure your child safely sleeps through the night.

Make sure you baby sleeps on his back. Your baby is much safer when he sleeps on his back than when he sleeps on his stomach or side. The mattress can actually smother your baby, especially if he or she cannot roll over.

Always lay your baby on his back.
You should also remind everyone who watches your baby to do the same – especially grandparents. This piece of advice didn't come out until 1994, which could be after you were raised. The risk of SIDS is also raised when a baby who is used to sleeping on his back is suddenly placed on his stomach.

Babies will not choke when they are on their backs like many people assume. If you are really concerned, like if your baby often coughs, you may ask your pediatrician if a special pillow will help.

When your baby hits 6-7 months, he will start rolling over on his own while he sleeps – you will have to allow it. However, since he can now roll, he is safer.

Purchase a firm bed and take out any soft toys or bedding. Your baby is more likely to suffocate with a soft cloth and mattresses. Make sure everything is firm, and don't use soft blankets, pillows, quilts, bumpers, or toys in the crib. Bumpers are allowed if you are able to keep the baby a good distance away from them.

If you have any questions about the safety of your mattress, you can talk to the Consumer Product Safety Commission.

Do not smoke around your baby. This is good advice all the way round, but particularly when it comes to SIDS. Babies who were born on women who smoked or children whose mother smoked while they were in the womb are 3 TIMES more likely to die from SIDS.

Don't let anyone smoke around your baby.

Try not to keep your baby in your bed – but keep him close. For whatever reason, studies show that babies who sleep in the same bed as their mother have a lower risk of SIDs. However, you might heighten the risk if you put him into your plush bed.

Never bring your baby into the bed with you when you're very tired or using medicines that affect your sleep.

Breastfeed for a long time.Breastfeeding is quite important for many aspects of your child's development. Studies have shown that breastfeeding can actually reduce your baby's risk of dying from SIDS by 50%.

Some theorize this is because breast milk protects babies from infections while others say that it is because the mother often keeps them close. Whatever the reason, do it.

Get your baby's shots. Babies who have been immunized properly and on schedule have a 50% reduced risk of dying from SIDS than those who aren't fully immunized.

Keep your baby nice and cool. Overheating is a possibility, especially with new parents who think that they need to keep the home really warm. Dress your baby in comfortable, light clothing. If the room is too warm for you, then the room is also too warm for the baby.

You are also better off purchasing a sleep sack rather than a blanket, which can put him in danger.

No matter what, go with your instincts and talk to your pediatrician if you have any questions or concerns.

TRIED AND TRUE METHODS

There have been quite a few different "waves" of sleep training that we have used in the last few decades. Is there one that is better than the others? Truthfully, it depends on the baby, the family, and the environment.

These are just the most popular, and there are many other sleep training methods that you can try – but we suggest that you start here to find what your baby likes the most.

Cry It Out

The Cry it Out Method is something that parents are divided upon, they either highly recommend or hate it. If it is something that you feel comfortable doing with your baby, there are two key things you need to know:

1.   It does not mean that you are denying your baby any form of comfort or affection;
2.   This method is harder on the parent than it is on the baby.

You are going to have a rough couple of nights when you are first starting out. Your instincts will tell you to go to your baby and help him or her. Instead, you have to let them cry it out, as the name suggests. Crying won't hurt your baby, nor will he remember any of this when he is older.

Can't stand it? Know that you are helping your baby learn how to sleep. Take turns if you can so that when it really gets to your heart, you can tap out.

Why it works: Those who believe in this method, including the most famous supporter, Dr. Ferber, know that by six months of age, babies are smart enough to know that crying will often allow them to be picked up, comforted, changed, rocked, or fed — which means that it is their first choice. However, once you break that habit, you will be able to see a change in behavior in just three or four nights!

How to make it work: You have to start while your baby is still awake. Put him into the crib, make sure he is safe, give him a kiss and tell him you love him and then leave the room. DO NOT wait until he is falling asleep. Especially at first, you can expect a lot of tears and cry. You might even hear some talking or babbling. Do yourself a favor and don't look at your video monitors. Wait until he has been crying for five minutes (time it) and then go in and say goodnight again. Every night, wait a little longer to go in and say goodnight again. Eventually, you will still hear crying, but it will only last a few moments.

How quickly it works: If you are looking for an instant result, this isn't the choice. It will take at least a week, but many people do see improvements after four nights. You won't hear the cries for too long, but it definitely takes a little bit of training – mostly for mom and dad!

Co-Sleeping

Co-sleeping is another option that is highly debatable among parents and doctors. Snuggling into bed with your baby might seem like one of the best and easiest things that you can do. However, some people do say that it is a bad idea. Now, in many parts of the world, this method is used by almost everyone. However, the American Academy of Pediatrics says that it can be dangerous.

Some research shows that co-sleeping leads to an increased risk for SIDS as well as the chance of suffocation from the parents and the bedding. The solution for co-sleeping, at least in the United States, is to sleep in the same bedroom, but not the same bed.

Why it works: This method allows the baby to learn how to fall asleep, but has the comfort of mom and/or dad at the same time. It cultivates independence while being easier for mom and dad to handle. In fact, most of these methods depend more on mom and dad than they do on the baby. However, a problem does arise because babies then get much more attached to mom and dad, and they may have trouble falling asleep without them around.

How to make it work: The best thing to do with this method is to start with your baby in your bed, but move him when he is just about asleep. Set his crib up near the bed, but try to keep at least a few feet between them. You want him to know you are there, but you want to foster independence while establishing this separation. Simply get your baby nearly to sleep, and then put him in the bed. Your presence will not only stop him from crying as soon as he is set down, but it will also allow him to sleep longer and better.

How quickly it works: This method works fairly well for the first year of life. However, as your baby gets older, you might want to move him. Not only does it create an incredibly specific environment that your baby needs to sleep, but it can also put a huge damper on your personal life.

Flexible Hours
A flexible hour sleeping is another method that many have used to lull their child to sleep without imposing boundaries. Some think that this might be one of the best ways to get a child to sleep without forcing any "trauma" on their minds.

This method works best for families where at least one parent stays home all the time, but it can also work for those who have flexible work schedules. It also helps with those babies that really cannot get on any sort of schedule.

The motto of this method is to just follow the baby.

Why it works: Flexible sleep scheduling works in a fairly straightforward way: you sleep when the baby sleeps. Now, you should try to have some sort of schedule in here as well. This method makes it so that you feel more rested which not only allows you to feel better, but will make your interactions with your baby much better. Flexible sleeping keeps everyone in line and helps to maximize the amount of sleep you get. However, a social and personal life may have to be sacrificed for a few months – until you can move your baby on to something else. This method is meant for younger babies, not toddlers.

How to make it work: Most families who find that flexible sleeping works when they start trying to put their baby to sleep at an earlier hour say 6 or 7 o'clock. Then, the parents themselves take a nap, wake up to get some personal time, and then the parents go back to sleep. You can still take turns to fight over who is going to stay up with the baby, and you can still try some of the other methods here as well. Just remember that you need to sleep when the baby is sleeping, or you only have yourself to blame if this doesn't work.

How quickly it works: The great thing about this method is that it works right away! You aren't changing any behaviors or breaking any bonds, instead, you are just going with the flow. If you want to try to slowly move your baby's schedule so that maybe he goes to bed a little later so that he sleeps for a longer block of time, that's all up to your scientific calculations.

Consistency

Your baby definitely needs to get some quality sleep -- but then again so do you! Establishing a proper baby sleep schedule that is consistent and follows rules is not just vital for the health, happiness, and well-being of the baby, but also for his parents, baby sitters, and just about anyone else who is around him all day.

You should be just as concerned; at least once your baby is home and safe, about maintaining consistency in sleeping and waking hours as you are about getting your baby to sleep.

How it works: As we have already talked about, your baby does not have any idea what lightness and darkness, or day and night really mean. They don't have a schedule programmed into their bodies yet – that is something that we learn. The goal of this method is to teach them about when the "proper" waking and sleeping hours are.

How to make it work: The first thing you need to do is teach your baby how to recognize day and night. Start as soon as the baby wakes up: get him dressed to symbolize a new day, be very active in the morning so that he knows this is an active time, feed him at consistent times and then develop a nighttime ritual. Start with a bath, soothing music, dimmed lights, and a book – whatever you want. You are essentially letting your baby know that this now the time to start settling down. Another key to making it work is to not focus on sleeping – this is a whole package type of deal. You will create eating, sleeping, changing, bathing, and even playing schedules. Want to schedule a little Mickey Mouse Clubhouse time? Go for it!

The most important thing you need to remember is those hours of sleep that babies need. Babies sleep a lot – of course, it is important to schedule hours for your baby to play and bond, but sleep is really what is most healthy. However, you can also look at it this way: the maximum time a baby can stay awake at a time and still get enough sleep:

• 0-6 weeks: 45 minutes

- 6-16 weeks: 60 to 80 minutes, depending
- 4-7 months: 90 to 150 minutes
- 7-12 months: 2 to 3 hours

How quickly it works: It may take a little while for your baby to get used to the method, but the key is to start right away. The best way to start is to go with a three-hour power cycle of eating, playing, and sleeping. If you do this, your baby will start to pick up the natural patterns: it is the way our brains are wired from the start! This isn't only good for the baby, but a good way for you to get used to the pattern, especially if you are breastfeeding.

How to maintain a schedule: Even if you aren't the type of person who typically likes a scheduled day, you will immediately start to see the rewards with this one. You will be able to get more done and plan out your day. Want to start exercising so that you can lose that baby weight? Want some grown up time? Schedule them! Want to be able to see that new movie, but you don't want your parents to have a grumpy baby? Pick a time when your baby is happiest.

Keep the schedule going, that's all you have to do. Sleeping, waking, and eating are so important, and they are really the only things your baby has to do for almost a year. Creating consistency is the best way to get through that year without any bumps in the road.

CREATING A SLEEPING PLAN

How exactly can you go and make a sleeping plan that will allow you to have a life and you aren't "going through the motions" as some new parents complain?

One of the biggest parts to creating a sleeping plan is that you cannot, under most circumstances, allow your baby to become overtired or overworked. Exhaustion is actually the root of all of the sleeping troubles that your baby (or you) may have.

While establishing a sleep schedule won't take away all of your problems, it will take away the root of many of them, a lack of sleep. These days are going to fly by, so you will want to make the most of them.

Creating the Plan

Although we know that babies vary in how much sleep they need, it is important that you take those numbers that we mentioned and stick them into your head. Print them out and put them on your refrigerator. Write them in lipstick on your bathroom mirror – do whatever you need. Skipping naps and causing your baby to miss too much sleep will result in him being irritable, having difficulty sleeping at night, and fighting off when it comes time for naps.

You have to first start to anticipate when your baby is going to sleep. You should watch and know when he's tired, as it won't be easy to see. Look at those signs that we pointed on in the first few chapters. Once you see the signs, you should break out the plan:

Step 1: Create a calm and tranquil environment about 20 minutes before bedtime.

Step 1 occurs when you can see the time, and then you can start to play with it. Go with your baby's body clock, but you can change it. Once you know the time, you can move it around by slowly shifting things a few minutes here or a few minutes there.

Step 2: Repetition
Once you have your plan, the only thing you really have to do is keep it. If you want to track it, you can log your results and keep everything down to the minute.

Why does this work?
Adequate rest leads to a healthier, happier and better behaved baby. Once he knows that there is a schedule, your baby will sleep and remain asleep because he feels comfortable.

You should know that when you are first putting your baby onto a schedule, the best approach is to let your baby cry it out. This is hard, but it is something that needs to happen to get him on the schedule. If you cuddle him to sleep, he won't understand that you are following a strict pattern.

If he wakes up in the middle of the night, try your best to rub him on the back and get him to sleep so that he stays on schedule.

Bonus Sleep Schedule Tip:
One of the best ways to get your baby used to the sleep schedule is to make sure that not only the times are the same, but the places are the same. Don't move around bathrooms, don't try to keep up the schedule while you are running errands, and keep your baby in his crib. Just try to stay at the moment.

DO's AND DO NOT's

To keep it short and simple, there are a few different things that you should definitely do to get a piece of mind when you are putting your baby to sleep or while he is sleeping.Some of these are facts that have been included

DO!

Put your baby into his crib so that he sleeps on his back. As you know, SIDS is a real threat no matter who you are, and the American Academy of Pediatrics recommends putting your baby on his back so that you can avoid that circumstance.

Dress him so that he is cool but still comfortable and cozy. Don't keep your baby too warm, or he will be uncomfortable. The rule of thumb is that his hands and feet should be cooler than the centermost part of his body. Aim to keep the room between 60-70 degrees.

Keep the room dark – try to avoid the nightlight. You want to teach your baby the difference between night and day and dark and light. Nightlights can have a negative impact on that.

Understand that your baby will wake up at night. So many people make a huge deal out of sleeping through the night, but you might not want that. If your baby is hungry, feed him!

DON'T

Be afraid to let your baby cry. Don't rush to every sound. You want to let your child learn independence from an early age. That might mean not keeping your baby monitors at the loudest level or not running to pick him up with every little whine or coo.

Rely on a pacifier as the only calming tool. Certainly, a pacifier has a place in your baby's life. However, getting him addicted to it will mean that you are going to be playing fetch with it, rinsing it off, and giving it back quite a few times a night.

Use soft bedding or pillows in the crib. Plush things can actually suffocate your baby or lead to SIDS.

Use the crib for anything other than sleeping. Some parents think of the crib as a place for baby to play while mommy cleans or a place to go when he behaved badly. Keep it a sleep only environment.

FAQ

When should my baby be able to start sleeping through the entire night without waking?

While we know that babies need to sleep many hours a day, sleep varies from one baby to another. They might have their days and nights mixed up or they might just get hungry a lot.

You shouldn't expect to see a full night's sleep until about 3-6 months of age. You will get longer uninterrupted times at least, sometimes stretching into 6-8 hours of sleep. Don't worry if your child isn't, however. That just means that he hasn't developed those skills yet.

If you are annoyed or need to get more sleep, try some of the methods we already mentioned in this book.

How can I get my baby to start sleeping through the night?

While it is definitely a system, you can start by keeping the room very dark and quiet. Start using a routine like we mentioned. Get him calm before you put him into a crib. Be consistent and work with her – not every day is going to be sunshine and rainbow.

The goal is to put your baby in his bed when he is drowsy because it means less crying and fussing, which can lead to an overtired baby and a harried parent.

If and when your baby wakes in the middle of the night, you should wait for a few minutes before checking in or peering into the room to see if he can fall back to sleep on his own. You can look in if he keeps crying, but try to let him cry it out. If your baby is awake but isn't crying, see if he can calm himself into going back to sleep. If the fussing continues, however, you may need to step in and help – your baby might be signaling something else.

How much nap time does my baby need?

It all really depends on how much your baby is sleeping at night. When babies are born, everything is eat, sleep, eat and sleep, so you don't really count any of that sleeping as naps. However, you should start to break the day down into patterns so that you can get in naps that last about 1.5 hours. Once your baby hits a year old, you can go down to one nap a day. By age 5, naps should disappear – don't worry; they'll come back when your baby goes to college.

Could my baby be waking up during the night because she's hungry?

After 4 months or so, you'll find that your baby probably won't need to eat as much during the night – unless he isn't eating as much during the day. Once again, you can move around this schedule if you need to.

Some babies just need to wake up and feed, then they'll go back to sleep. Instead of denying the feeding, and having the crying, it's best to feed him and move on – you will thank yourself for it in the morning.

CONCLUSION

Getting sleep with a new baby in your life isn't the easiest thing. However, you have to remember that now you must do what is best for your baby. That means that you might have to go outside of your own comfort zone and do something things that you might not normally do.

If getting enough sleep at night means that you have to go to bed at 7 PM and miss your favorite television show, so be it. That's why they invented Netflix.

Instead of focusing on the bad things and how tired you are, instead focus on how you are changing the world simply by creating this little one and all of the magic that he brings.

Good night, sleep tight, and don't let those bed bugs bite!

Finally, if you enjoyed this book, please click below to share your thoughts and post a positive review on Amazon. I would greatly appreciate your support!

Thank you and good luck!

Sarah Rene

ADDITIONAL RESOURCES

Please point your web browser to **www.plaid-enterprises.com** for more related resources, my full bibliography and to grab your FREE book!